Calming Inflammation

7 Tested Techniques for Immune Balance, Gut Wellness, Stress Reduction, and Optimal Living

Virgie W. Miller

COPYRIGHT

TABLE OF CONTENTS

Calming Inflammation

Calming Inflammation

Calming Inflammation

Calming Inflammation

INTRODUCTION

Have you ever experienced the swelling from a sprained ankle, the redness of a sunburn, or the heat of a fever? All of them indicate inflammation, which is your body's first line of defense against damage and infection. It's a common experience, a shared indication that something within us is off.

Because inflammation has two sides, it's a serious health concern. When it's acute, it's vital for healing; but, when it's persistent, it can subtly aggravate a variety of illnesses. Consider a security system that is perpetually on high alert, leading to more harm than benefit over time. That's chronic inflammation, an overactive immune response that can harm the body's tissues and result in autoimmune diseases, heart disease, arthritis, and other ailments.

Chronic inflammation has a significant and wide-ranging effect. It can reduce our longevity, impact our long-term health, and change how we feel daily. However, hope remains. We may reduce the negative impacts of chronic inflammation and enhance our general health by being aware of it and taking appropriate action.

We will examine seven tried-and-true methods in this book that provide a break from the never-ending flood of inflammation. These tactics are not merely theoretical; they are useful, approachable, and have been shown to have an impact. Among them are:

Immune Balance: regulating the immune system to keep it from becoming too active.

Gut Wellness: Taking care of the bacteria in the gut, which is essential for controlling inflammation.

Stress Reduction: Reducing the body's inflammatory reaction brought on by stress by using stress management practices.

Anti-Inflammatory Diet: Selecting nourishing but naturally anti-inflammatory foods.

Physical Activity: Regular exercise can improve health and lower inflammatory indicators.

Holistic Approaches: Including complementary therapies such as massage and acupuncture to assist the body's inherent healing abilities.

Lifestyle Modifications: Modifying daily routines in a sustainable, minor way can significantly lower inflammation levels.

Every method is a step toward a healthier, more balanced condition of mind and body. They aim to create a lifestyle that supports and maintains a body in harmony, not only to suppress symptoms. We will explore each strategy in detail, learn about the research underlying it, hear from others who have benefited, and discover how to incorporate it into our lives for the best possible quality of life.

CHAPTER 1

AN INTRODUCTION TO INFLAMMATION

Inflammation: The Rapid Reaction of the Body to Damage

The word "inflammation" frequently evokes thoughts of pain, swelling, and redness. It is the natural reaction of the body to an inflammatory, pathogenic, or damaged stimuli. By eliminating the damaging stimuli and starting the healing process, the body is attempting to defend itself.

There are two primary categories of inflammation: acute and chronic. The first reaction to an injury or infection is known as acute inflammation. The characteristic symptoms of redness, heat, swelling, discomfort, and loss of function are what define it. This kind of inflammation usually passes after a few days. Chronic inflammation may develop from acute inflammation if the underlying cause is not addressed.

An extended inflammatory response that lasts for months or years is known as chronic inflammation. It's a more covert and sneaky process that frequently goes unrecognized until it takes the form of different illnesses. Persistent infections, extended exposure to irritants, autoimmune reactions, and obesity are all known to cause chronic inflammation.

Providing Examples of the Inflammatory Process

To better understand the inflammatory process, consider how the body might react to a typical finger splinter. A splinter punctures the skin, causing microorganisms to enter and destroy cells. When the immune system perceives something as dangerous, an inflammatory reaction is triggered by the body. To bring white blood cells and other immune cells to the location to combat the germs and start tissue repair, blood vessels widen. The redness and swelling we see are indicative of this response.

Chronic Inflammation: An Imperceptible Danger

Although it is significantly more hazardous, chronic inflammation is less noticeable than acute inflammation. It resembles an ongoing low-grade fever. This constant alertness has the potential to cause tissue damage over time and accelerate the onset of conditions like cancer, diabetes, and heart disease.

Patient Testimonials: The Inflammatory Human Side

To illustrate the idea of chronic inflammation, let's look at 42-year-old Maria, a teacher who spent years dealing with unexplained lethargy, stomach problems, and joint discomfort. She was diagnosed with persistent inflammation as a result of an autoimmune illness after multiple medical visits. Maria's path to managing her inflammation involved medication, dietary adjustments, and stress reduction; this illustrates the multimodal approach required to address chronic inflammation.

CHAPTER 2

DEFENSE AGAINST INFECTION

The Immune System's Fundamentals

When the immune system is in balance, it protects the body from infectious infections as effectively as possible without overreacting and creating allergies or autoimmune conditions. To stay healthy and avoid infections and chronic diseases, this balance is essential.

Lifestyle Selections to Modulate Immune Response

Lifestyle Selections to Modulate Immune Response

Numerous factors, such as stress levels, sleep patterns, physical exercise, and nutrition, have an impact on the immune system. Adopting a lifestyle that promotes the immune system's healthy functioning is crucial for immune system modulation. This entails using mindfulness techniques to manage stress, getting enough restful sleep, exercising frequently, abstaining from tobacco use, and consuming little to no alcohol.

Nutritional Decisions to Boost Immune Function

Our immune system's functioning is significantly influenced by the foods we eat. Immune equilibrium can be preserved with an anti-inflammatory diet high in fruits, vegetables,

Calming Inflammation

whole grains, lean protein, and healthy fats. Berries, nuts, leafy greens, and fatty fish are among the foods that are well-known for their anti-inflammatory qualities.

Foods and Supplements Anti-Inflammatory

The following is an inventory of foods and substances that reduce inflammation and have been proven to do so by science:

Turmeric: This spice has curcumin, a powerful anti-inflammatory.

Ginger: renowned for its antioxidant and anti-inflammatory qualities.

Omega-3 Fatty Acids: These can help lower inflammation and are present in flaxseed and fish oil.

Vitamin D: Found in supplements and meals enriched with nutrients, it supports the immune system.

Probiotics: They support a healthy gut microbiome and are present in yogurt and fermented meals.

Including Immune-Supportive Activities in Everyday Life

Start small when implementing these immune-supportive habits into your everyday routine. Find an activity you enjoy and can commit to regularly, arrange normal sleep hours, and include a dish of anti-inflammatory foods in each meal. To acquire stress-reduction methods and incorporate them into your daily practice, think about taking mindfulness courses or using apps.

CHAPTER 3

HEALTH OF THE GUT

The Gut's Fundamental Function in General Health

Often referred to as the body's "second brain," the stomach is essential to general health. It is in charge of breaking down food, taking in nutrients, and releasing waste. However, its impact goes well beyond simple digestion. The gut, which is home to a huge network of bacteria known as the gut microbiome, is also a vital component of the immune system.

The link between the Immune System and Gut Microbiota

Trillions of bacteria, viruses, and fungi make up this microbiome, which is present in the gastrointestinal tract and coexists there. A balanced gut flora is necessary for a healthy immune system.It contributes to the synthesis of certain vitamins, controls inflammation, and provides defense against infections.

Keeping the Gut Flora Healthy

To lower inflammation, a healthy gut flora community is essential. Increased intestinal permeability, sometimes known as "leaky gut," is a result of dysbiosis, an imbalance that can allow bacteria and toxins to enter the circulation and perhaps cause inflammation throughout the body.

Calming Inflammation

Encouraging the good bacteria and suppressing the bad ones are key to improving gut health. A diet high in fiber, which functions as a prebiotic and feeds the good bacteria, can help achieve this, as can consuming fermented foods that contain probiotics, or the beneficial bacteria themselves.

Fermented Foods and a Diet High in Fibre

Probiotic-rich foods include yogurt, kefir, sauerkraut, and kombucha. Whole grains, legumes, fruits, and vegetables are examples of foods high in fiber. These meals provide vital nutrients and lower inflammation, which improve general health in addition to promoting the gut microbiota.

This is a straightforward menu to promote intestinal health:

Greek yogurt for **breakfast** topped with a mixture of berries and chia seeds.

Lunch consists of quinoa salad dressed with lemon-tahini dressing, avocado, chickpeas, and mixed greens.

Snack: Almond butter on sliced apples.

Dinner is brown rice and grilled salmon served with a side of steamed broccoli.

Dessert: A tiny piece of dark chocolate, as it has antioxidants called polyphenols that are good for the flora in the stomach.

Recipe for Probiotic Smoothie

Ingredients

- A single cup of kefir or simple yogurt

- 1/2 cup of blueberries, frozen

- One banana

- A handful of spinach leaves

- One tablespoon honey (optional)

Guidelines

- Enjoy a tasty, stomach-friendly smoothie after blending all ingredients until smooth.

Recipe for Fiber-Rich Lentil Soup

Ingredients

- One tablespoon of olive oil

- One chopped onion

- Two diced carrots

Calming Inflammation

- Two celery stalks, chopped
- Two minced garlic cloves
- One cup of washed lentils
- 1 can of chopped tomatoes
- 4 cups vegetable broth
- 1 teaspoon each of cumin and coriander
- To taste, add salt and pepper.

Guidelines

- In olive oil, sauté the onion, carrots, celery, and garlic until they become tender.
- Stir in the tomatoes, spices, broth, and lentils.
- Once the lentils are soft, simmer them.
- Add pepper and salt for seasoning.

Healthy Berry Smoothie

Guidelines

- One banana
- One cup of mixed berries (strawberries, raspberries, and blueberries)
- One spoonful of chia seeds and one cup of spinach leaves
- One cup of kefir or almond milk
- A honey drizzle (not required)

Guidelines

- Mix every item until it's smooth. This smoothie is a great option for a gut-friendly breakfast or snack because it's loaded with fiber, probiotics, and antioxidants.

Quinoa & Roasted Vegetable Salad

Ingredients

- 1 cup quinoa, 2 cups water
- 1 chopped bell pepper
- 1 chopped zucchini
- 1 chopped red onion
- 2 tablespoons olive oil
- 1 tablespoon balsamic vinegar
- salt, and pepper to taste
- fresh herbs for garnish (such cilantro or parsley)

Guidelines

- To cook the quinoa, follow the instructions on the package.In the meantime,
- combine olive oil, salt, and pepper with the zucchini, bell pepper, and red onion

- Roast at 400°F (200°C) in a preheated oven until soft and beginning to caramelize.

- Toss with the cooked quinoa, add the roasted veggies, and sprinkle with the fresh herbs and balsamic vinegar.

Probiotic-Rich Berry Yogurt Bowl

Ingredients

- One cup of probiotic-rich Greek yogurt
- ½ cup of mixed berries, including strawberries, blueberries, and raspberries
- One tablespoon of chia seeds, which are a great fiber source
- One spoonful of honey, for sweetness naturally
- A small handful of almonds (for their healthful fats and crunch)

Guidelines

- Pour the Greek yogurt into a bowl.
- Sprinkle mixed berries evenly over the yogurt and top.
- Add almonds and chia seeds to the top.
- Pour some honey into the bowl to provide a little sweetness.
- Savor this dish as a healthy way to start the day!

Cool Cucumber Avocado Salad
Ingredients

- Diced two medium cucumbers
- One sliced ripe avocado
- 1/2 thinly sliced red onion
- 1/4 cup finely chopped fresh cilantro
- One lime's juice
- Two tsp extra virgin olive oil
- To taste, add salt and pepper.

Guidelines:

- Combine the red onion, avocado, and cucumbers in a big bowl.
- Fill the bowl with the chopped cilantro.
- In a small bowl, mix the lime juice, olive oil, salt, and pepper.
- Drizzle the salad with the dressing and toss to coat.
- You may either serve right away or chill in the fridge before serving.

Filling Soup with Lentil and Veggies

Ingredients

- 1 tablespoon olive oil
- 1 chopped onion
- 2 minced garlic cloves
- 2 sliced carrots
- Two celery stalks, chopped
- One cup of washed dried lentils
- One can (14.5 oz) chopped tomatoes

- 2 cups spinach leaves
- 1 teaspoon each of dried thyme and ground cumin
- 6 cups vegetable broth - Salt and pepper to taste

Guidelines:
- Heat the olive oil in a big pot over medium heat. Add the garlic and onion, and cook until they become tender.
- Cook for a further five minutes after adding the carrots and celery.
- Add the cumin, thyme, diced tomatoes, vegetable broth, and lentils. Heat till boiling.
- Simmer the lentils for about 30 minutes, or until they are soft, on low heat with a lid on.
- Season with salt and pepper, to taste.

Calming Inflammation

- Include the spinach leaves and simmer for two minutes, or until wilted.
- If desired, top with a sprinkle of fresh herbs and serve hot.

Savor these meals as a part of a well-balanced diet to help maintain intestinal health!

CHAPTER 4

REDUCING STRESS

The Relationship Between Inflammation and Stress

Stress has significant medical effects as well as psychological ones, especially when it comes to inflammation. Stress triggers our body's "fight-or-flight" reaction, which causes the release of adrenaline and cortisol. Even if these hormones are helpful in brief spurts, long-term stress causes a persistent release of these hormones, which can then cause inflammation all across the body. Numerous medical conditions, including arthritis and heart disease, can be exacerbated by this inflammation.

Numerous methods are successful in reducing the effects of stress, including:

Meditation: Meditation can assist in bringing the mind into focus and lowering the flow of ideas that cause stress. It's a short practice that takes place anywhere and can help you feel at ease in a matter of minutes.

Yoga: This holistic method of reducing stress combines physical postures, breathing techniques, and meditation. It also helps to quiet the mind and enhances strength, flexibility, and balance.

Deep-Breathing Exercises: These easy-to-do but effective breathing techniques can help trigger the body's relaxation response, which lowers blood pressure and slows heart rate.

Gradual Relaxation of the Muscles

This entails beginning at your toes and working your way up to tensing and then relaxing each muscle group in your body. It can promote relaxation and increase your awareness of your body's sensations.

Exercise: One of the best strategies to reduce stress is to engage in regular physical activity. Exercise can make you feel happier, sleep better, and have more energy. Exercises like cycling, swimming, jogging, and walking can be very advantageous.

Social Assistance

Maintaining relationships with friends and family can help you cope with stress and offer emotional support. Speaking with a trusted person about your worries and emotions can be incredibly beneficial.

Calming Inflammation

Time Administration

By giving you control over your schedule and responsibilities, effective time management can help you feel less stressed. Setting objectives, assigning responsibilities, and prioritizing your activities will all help you manage your workload more effectively.

Gratitude in Self-Talk

Changing your perspective on stress can have a significant impact on your mental health. Consider problems as chances for progress rather than as threats.

Interests and Artistic endeavors

Taking up enjoyable hobbies or artistic pursuits can be a terrific way to decompress and remove yourself from stressful situations. Find something to do that makes you happy,

Calming Inflammation

whether it's writing, painting, gardening, or playing music.

Using aromatherapy

Stress and anxiety can be lessened by using scented candles or essential oils. Particularly calming smells include sandalwood, chamomile, and lavender.

Always keep in mind that what works for one person might not work for another, so it's critical to identify the stress-reduction strategies that are most effective for you. See which of these tactics makes you feel more at ease and in control when you try implementing a handful of them into your daily routine.

A healthy sleep schedule is essential for managing stress. The body heals itself as we sleep, strengthening memories and replenishing vitality. Stress can be made worse by sleep deprivation, which can lead to a vicious cycle of rising anxiety and falling asleep. To enhance one's sleeping habits:

Establish a Calm Environment: Make sure your bedroom is cold, quiet, and dark. To block light and muffle sound, use blackout curtains or eye masks, and use white noise generators.

Create a Routine: To help your body's internal clock to function properly, go to bed and wake up at the same time every day.

Watch Your Nutrition: Since they can interfere with sleep, avoid caffeine and large meals right before bed.

Calming Inflammation

Creating a relaxation practice is a great way to reduce stress. Here's a quick routine to get you going:

Locate a Quiet Space: Decide on a location where you won't be bothered.

Start with Deep Breathing: To tell your body to relax, take calm, deep breaths.

Progressive Muscle Relaxation: Tend each muscle group from your toes to your head, then release it.

Visualization: Envision a serene setting, concentrating on the specifics and feelings of this secure area.

Being mindful Meditation: Pay attention to the here and now, recognizing and releasing thoughts as they come to you.

Calming Inflammation

Gentle Stretching: To relieve any last bits of tension in your body, stretch a little bit at the end of your workout.

Journaling: Take a few minutes to jot down your ideas or consider the day that has passed. This can help you decompress and reduce any residual tension.

Aromatherapy: To create a relaxing ambiance, add smells like lavender or chamomile.

Warm beverage: To help your body relax and let you know when it's time to wind down, sip on a warm, non-caffeinated beverage like herbal tea.

Reflection on Gratitude: Take a moment to list or consider the things for which you are thankful. This uplifting thought might change your perspective and ease your tension.

Gentle Yoga: To stretch out your body and relieve tension, try a few gentle yoga poses.

Calming Inflammation

Walking with awareness: If at all feasible, go for a stroll while paying attention to your surroundings and how each step feels.

These actions can be included in your everyday routine to help control stress and foster peace of mind and overall well-being. Recall that finding what works best for you and being consistent are the keys to a successful relaxing regimen. Please feel free to modify these recommendations to suit your tastes and way of life.

CHAPTER 5

ANTI-INFLAMMATORY DIET

An Anti-Inflammatory Diet's
Fundamentals

Eating foods that are known to lower inflammation while avoiding those that can increase it is the goal of an anti-inflammatory diet. This diet is based on the same principles as the Mediterranean diet, with an emphasis on full, nutrient-dense foods. Important elements consist of:

Calming Inflammation

Fruits and vegetables: Packed with phytonutrients and antioxidants that help fight inflammation.

Whole Grains: Offer vital minerals and fiber.

Nuts, avocados, and olive oil are good sources of **healthy fats**.

Lean Proteins: These come from plant-based foods like beans and seafood.

Herbs and Spices: Anti-inflammatory qualities are well-known for garlic, ginger, and turmeric.

Additional foods that reduce inflammation and their purposes include the following:

Berries: Anthocyanins, which are antioxidants, are found in berries such as raspberries, blackberries, blueberries, and strawberries. The anti-inflammatory properties of these substances may lower the chance of illness.

Saturated Fish: Omega-3 fatty acids, specifically eicosapentaenoic acid (EPA) and docosahexaenoic acid (DHA), are abundant in fatty fish, including salmon, sardines, herring, mackerel, and anchovies. These fats have been connected to a lower risk of chronic diseases and can help reduce inflammation.

Broccoli: A cruciferous vegetable, broccoli is rich in nutrients and linked to a lower risk of cancer and heart disease. Sulforaphane, an anti-inflammatory antioxidant, is present in it.

Avocados: Avocados are high in heart-healthy monounsaturated fats, fiber, potassium, and magnesium. They also include tocopherols and carotenoids, which have been connected to a lower risk of cancer.

Green Tea: Studies have demonstrated that the antioxidant epigallocatechin gallate (EGCG), which is abundant in green tea, can lower inflammation and shield cells from deterioration.

Chilis: Rich in antioxidants and vitamin C, bell and chili peppers have potent anti-inflammatory properties.

Mushrooms: Despite their wide variety, mushrooms are rich in selenium, copper, and all the B vitamins and low in calories. They also have additional antioxidants, such as phenols, which offer protection against inflammation.

Grapes: The anthocyanins found in grapes have anti-inflammatory properties. Additionally, they may lower the chance of developing several illnesses, such as diabetes, obesity, heart disease, Alzheimer's, and eye problems.

Turmeric: Curcumin, a potent anti-inflammatory ingredient found in turmeric, has drawn a lot of attention. Because it increases the absorption of curcumin, black pepper and turmeric work best together.

Extra Virgin Olive Oil: Of all the fats in your diet, extra virgin olive oil is one of the healthiest. It is a mainstay of the anti-inflammatory Mediterranean diet and is high in monounsaturated fats. Heart disease, brain tumors, and other significant health disorders may be less likely to occur if olive oil is used.

Cocoa with Dark Chocolate: Antioxidants like flavonoids, which are abundant in dark chocolate, may help lower inflammation. To get the benefits, it's critical to select dark chocolate with at least 70% cocoa content.

Tomatoes: Tomatoes are rich in potassium, vitamin C, and the antioxidant lycopene, which has strong anti-inflammatory qualities.

Cherries: Antioxidants found in cherries, such as anthocyanins and catechins, may be useful in the fight against inflammation. Studies have demonstrated the health benefits of both sweet and sour cherries.

Nuts: Good fats found in almonds, walnuts, and other nuts can help reduce inflammation.

Including these foods in your diet will help you feel better overall and minimize inflammation. Recall that you should also cut back on or completely avoid items that can aggravate inflammation, such as processed meals, refined carbohydrates, and unhealthy fats. These foods should not just be included in your diet. It's ideal to consistently include a variety of these anti-inflammatory foods in a healthy diet for a balanced approach.

Foods to stay away from

It's crucial to understand which meals to restrict or stay away from to lessen inflammation:

Refined carbohydrates, which can exacerbate inflammation, including those found in white bread and pastries.

Fried foods: Trans fats, which cause inflammation, may be present in them.

Sugary Drinks: Inflammation may be exacerbated by soda and other sweetened beverages.

Red meat and processed meats: Inflammation levels have been related to foods like sausages, hot dogs, burgers, and steaks.

Changing Your Diet to Be Less Inflammatory

Due to its strong adherence to the principles of anti-inflammatory food, the Mediterranean diet is frequently advised. It has an abundance of whole grains, seafood, nuts, fruits, veggies, and healthy oils. Maintaining this diet consistently can help lower the risk of inflammatory-related chronic disorders.

Recall that the objective is to develop a varied and balanced diet that minimizes foods that can aggravate inflammation while including a range of anti-inflammatory foods. Making healthy decisions that can support long-term well-being is more important than striving for perfection.

The Science of Foods That Reduce Inflammation

Anti-inflammatory foods include those high in omega-3 fatty acids and antioxidants. While omega-3 fatty acids help limit the creation of chemicals and substances connected to inflammation, antioxidants help lower levels of free radicals, which can promote inflammation

Sweet Potato and Chickpea Stew

A satisfying stew that is suitable for any time of year.

Ingredients

- 1 can rinsed and drained chickpeas
- 1 large chopped onion
- 2 minced garlic cloves
- 1 large peeled and cubed sweet potato
- 1/2 tsp cayenne pepper (adjust to taste)
- 1 tsp ground cumin
- One can of chopped tomatoes
- Four cups of vegetable broth
- Season with salt and pepper
- Garnish with fresh cilantro

Guidelines:

- Heat the olive oil in a big pot over medium heat. Add the garlic and onion and sauté until transparent.
- Include the chickpeas, cumin, cayenne, and sweet potato cubes. After combining, cook for two minutes.
- Add the veggie broth and diced tomatoes. After bringing to a boil, lower the heat, and cook the sweet potatoes until they are soft, about 20 minutes.
- To taste, add salt and pepper for seasoning.
- Add some fresh cilantro as a garnish and serve hot.

Calming Inflammation

A salad of kale and quinoa dressed with lemon

A nutrient-rich, light, and pleasant salad.

Ingredients:

- 2 cups cooked, cooked quinoa
- 4 cups chopped, stem-free kale
- 1/2 cup toasted almond slices
- 1/2 cup crumbled feta cheese
- diced cucumber
- 1/4 cup extra virgin olive oil
- One lemon's juice
- One tablespoon of honey
- To taste, add salt and pepper.

Guidelines:

- Put the cooked quinoa, diced cucumber, feta cheese, chopped kale, and toasted almonds in a big bowl.

- Combine the olive oil, lemon juice, and honey in a small bowl. Add pepper and salt for seasoning.

- Drizzle the salad with the dressing and toss to evenly coat.

- To allow the flavors to mingle, let the salad sit for ten minutes before serving.

Ginger-Turmeric Salmon

Ingredients:

- 2 tsp turmeric powder
- 4 salmon filets
- 1 tsp grated ginger and 1 tbsp olive oil
- To taste, add salt and pepper
- Serve with lemon wedges

Guidelines

- Set the oven temperature to 375°F or 190°C.
- Combine olive oil, salt, and pepper with ginger and turmeric.
- Coat the salmon filets with the mixture.
- Arrange the filets on a parchment paper-lined baking sheet.
- Bake for 15 to 20 minutes, or until a fork can easily pierce the salmon.
- Present with wedges of lemon.

Black bean and avocado salad

Ingredients

- Diced two ripe avocados
- Rinsed and drained can of black bean
- Diced red bell pepper
- 1/4 cup finely chopped red onion
- 1/4 cup finely chopped fresh cilantro
- One lime's juice

- Two tablespoons of extra virgin olive oil

- To taste, add salt and pepper.

Guidelines:

- Combine bell pepper, red onion, black beans, and avocados in a big bowl.

- In a small bowl, mix together lime juice, olive oil, salt, and pepper.

- Drizzle the salad with the dressing and toss to mix lightly.

- Before serving, garnish with fresh cilantro.

Anti-Inflammatory Smoothie

Ingredients

- 1/2 cup frozen blueberries

- 1 cup spinach

- One half banana

- One tablespoon of flaxseeds

- 1 teaspoon ground turmeric

- 1 cup almond milk

- 1/2 tsp grated ginger

Directions:

- Put all the ingredients in a blender.

- Process until smooth.

- For a revitalizing and anti-inflammatory boost, serve right away.

Roasted Cauliflower Soup

Ingredients

- 1 head of cauliflower, chopped into florets

- Two tablespoons of olive oil

- One chopped onion;

- Two minced garlic cloves

- One teaspoon of cumin

- Four cups of vegetable broth

- Season with salt and pepper

- Garnish with fresh parsley

Calming Inflammation

Directions

- Set the oven's temperature to 425°F (220°C).
- Combine 1 tablespoon olive oil, salt, and pepper with the cauliflower florets.
- Roast until brown and soft, about 25 minutes.
- Place the remaining olive oil in a pot and warm it over medium heat. Add the chopped garlic and onion, and cook until they are soft and transparent.
- Include the roasted cauliflower in the pot with the cumin and vegetable broth.
- Bring to a boil, then simmer for 20 minutes on low heat.
- Puree the soup with an immersion blender until it's smooth. To taste, add salt and pepper for seasoning.
- Garnish with fresh parsley and serve hot.

Calming Inflammation

Mango salsa served with grilled chicken

Ingredients

- Four skinless, boneless chicken breasts
- One chopped ripe mango
- Half a diced red bell pepper
- 1/4 cup finely chopped red onion
- 1 minced and seeded jalapeño
- One lime's juice
- 1 tablespoon olive oil
- 2 tablespoons chopped fresh cilantro
- Salt and pepper to taste

Directions

- Set the grill's temperature to medium-high.
- Apply a light coating of olive oil and season chicken breasts with salt and pepper.

Calming Inflammation

- Cook the chicken on the grill for 6–7 minutes on each side, or until done.
- Combine mango, lime juice, cilantro, jalapeño, red bell pepper, and red onion in a bowl. Add pepper and salt for seasoning.
- Present the grilled chicken with a dollop of raw mango salsa on top.

An Anti-Inflammatory Meal Plan for a Week

Day 1:

Almond milk and blueberries with oatmeal for **breakfast**.

Quinoa salad with mixed veggies and a dressing made of olive oil for **lunch**.

Steamed broccoli and sweet potatoes paired with grilled fish for **dinner**.

Day 2:

Greek yogurt with walnuts and honey for **breakfast**.

Lentil soup and mixed greens on the side for **lunch**.

The **supper** consists of brown rice, roasted Brussels sprouts, and baked chicken.

Day 3

Banana, spinach, and flaxseed smoothie for **breakfast**.

Turkey wrap with sprouts and avocado for **lunch**.

Quinoa and bell peppers with stir-fried tofu for **dinner**.

Day 4

Eggs scrambled with spinach and mushrooms for **breakfast**.

Chickpea salad with cucumber, tomatoes, and feta cheese for **lunch**.

Baked cod served with barley and asparagus for **dinner**.

Day 5

Mixed berry and chia seed pudding for **breakfast.**

Brown rice and vegetable stir-fry for **lunch**.

Pasta tossed with tomato sauce and a side salad for **dinner**.

Day 6

Avocado and whole grain toast for **breakfast**.

Cornbread and black bean soup for **lunch**.

Dinner is quinoa, green beans, and roasted turkey breast.

Day 7

Oat flour pancakes with fresh fruit on top for **breakfast.**

Lunch consists of whole grain bread and caprese salad.

Dinner is farro and grilled shrimp with a variety of veggies.

Moderation and Consistency in Dietary Decisions

Eating wholesome meals regularly can help reduce cravings and the risk of overindulging. Eating a variety of foods to maintain a balance of nutrients and ingesting the appropriate amount of food to suit the body's demands are both examples of moderation.

CHAPTER 6

INFLAMMATION AND PHYSICAL ACTIVITY

Towards Well-Being: The Function of Exercise in Inflammation Control

A healthy lifestyle is generally attributed to physical activity, which has several advantages for the body and mind. However, did you know that exercise is also essential for reducing inflammation and enhancing general well-being? Frequent physical activity has been demonstrated to have potent anti-inflammatory effects that can help control inflammation, from lowering levels of pro-inflammatory cytokines to enhancing immunological function.

Our bodies go through several physiological changes while we exercise, which have an effect on inflammation on several levels. Exercise has an important role in modulating inflammation through its effects on body fat, or adipose tissue. Not only is adipose tissue a passive store of energy, but it is also an active endocrine organ that releases and generates inflammatory cytokines including interleukin-6 (IL-6) and tumor necrosis factor-alpha (TNF-alpha).

Frequent exercise aids in the reduction of visceral adipose tissue, the kind of fat most closely linked to inflammation and the risk of chronic illness. Pro-inflammatory cytokine production falls with body fat, resulting in a more balanced inflammatory profile and reduced systemic inflammation.

Exercise has also been demonstrated to increase the synthesis of anti-inflammatory cytokines, such as interleukin-10 (IL-10), which assist in reducing inflammation and encourage the regeneration and repair of damaged tissue. Exercise supports a change toward a more anti-inflammatory state, which balances the immune system and lowers the risk of diseases linked to chronic inflammation.

Exercises That Work Well for Controlling Inflammation

It has been found that the following types of exercise are very beneficial in reducing inflammation:

Aerobic Exercise: Exercises that raise the heart rate and enhance oxygen utilization by the body, such as walking, cycling, and swimming, can help lower inflammation.

Resistance Training: Using resistance bands or lifting weights increases muscular growth and strength, which can reduce inflammation brought on by aging and muscle atrophy.

Yoga and Pilates: These physical activities emphasize strength, flexibility, and breathing, all of which might help lessen inflammation brought on by stress.

High-Intensity Interval Training (HIIT): Research has demonstrated that brief bursts of vigorous exercise, interspersed with rest intervals, can lower markers of inflammation.

These are some more targeted stretches or workouts that reduce inflammation:

Calming Inflammation

Yoga To lower stress and inflammation, yoga incorporates breathing techniques, postures, and meditation. Because of its emphasis on relaxing and stretching, it's especially advantageous.

Aqua aerobics and Swimming

Exercises done in the water are easy on the joints and can be a fantastic way to keep active while putting less strain on your body. The impact of movements is lessened by the buoyancy of water.

Aerobic Dancing: Dancing is a great method to reduce tension in the body and encourage healing. It's also enjoyable. It's a terrific way to add moderate-intensity exercise to your regimen and can cause an anti-inflammatory reaction.

Calming Inflammation

Strolling: Walking is a straightforward yet powerful kind of exercise that can reduce inflammation, increase energy, and enhance memory. It's widely available and has a lot of health advantages.

Resistance Training: By utilizing weights or resistance bands, resistance training can help increase muscle mass and strength, which is crucial for reducing the inflammation brought on by aging.

Extending: Stretching regularly helps increase circulation and flexibility, which may help lower inflammation. It's a low-impact exercise that you may perform whenever and wherever you choose.

Tai chi: Deep breathing and slow motions are hallmarks of this mild style of martial arts, which can help lower inflammation and stress.

Pilates: Pilates aims to improve physical function and reduce inflammation by emphasizing flexibility, strength, and conscious movement.

Including these workouts in your regimen can assist with inflammation management. It's critical to select enjoyable and anticipated activities because they will support you in keeping up a regular exercise routine. Furthermore, pay attention to your body's needs at all times and modify the length and intensity of your workouts to fit your fitness level and unique requirements. Before beginning a new exercise program, it's a good idea to speak with a healthcare physician or a fitness professional if you're new to exercising or if you have any health problems.

This is an example of a week-long fitness plan that includes a range of exercises:

Monday

Walk briskly for thirty minutes in the **morning**; perform 20 minutes of weight training in the **evening**.

Tuesday

Swimming for thirty minutes in the morning
Evening: yoga session

Wednesday

20 minutes of HIIT in the **morning**
Pilates session in the **evening**

Thursday

Take a day off from work and engage in some gentle stretching and strolling.

Friday

30 minutes of cycling in the **morning**

20 minutes of weight training in the **evening**

Saturday

Morning: Group exercise session outside

Evening: Yoga poses for relaxation

Sunday

Leisure day with the ability to engage in modest exercise, such as walking or recreational sports

Overcoming Obstacles to Physical Activity

Exercise is frequently impeded by a lack of time, energy, enthusiasm, or fear of injury. Here are a few ways to overcome these obstacles:

Lack of Time: Set out certain times in your calendar for physical activity, and opt for activities that you can incorporate into your everyday routine, such as taking a stroll during lunch breaks.

Lack of Motivation: Find a training partner or group to hold you accountable, track your progress, and set clear goals.

Lack of Energy: Plan your workouts for when you're at your most alert and don't forget that physical activity increases your energy.

Fear of Injuries: Begin with low-impact workouts and progressively up the ante. To guarantee correct technique, think about collaborating with a fitness expert.

CHAPTER 7

ALL-ENCOMPASSING METHODS

Overview of Integrative and Holistic Therapies for the Management of Inflammation

The whole person—body, mind, and spirit—is taken into account when addressing health and wellness in holistic and integrative therapies. Instead of only treating the symptoms of inflammation, they seek to maximize health by addressing its underlying causes. These therapies cover a broad spectrum of treatments, from conventional methods like massage and acupuncture to dietary adjustments and stress reduction.

Calming Inflammation

Acupuncture: Studies have revealed which neurons are necessary for acupuncture to cause an anti-inflammatory reaction. Research indicates that in several diseases, acupuncture may be able to lessen systemic inflammation.

Massage: It is well known that massage therapy helps people relax and feel less stressed, both of which can help control inflammation. Although there is still a lack of conclusive research, preliminary studies and anecdotal reports indicate that massage reduces inflammation.

Herbal therapy: For ages, herbal therapy has been used to treat a wide range of illnesses, including inflammation. Strong anti-inflammatory qualities can be found in bioactive chemicals found in herbs such as green tea, Boswellia, turmeric, and ginger. You may naturally boost immunological balance and reduce inflammation by including these herbs in your diet or utilizing them as supplements.

Mindfulness and Meditation: Deep breathing, guided imagery, and mindfulness exercises all encourage relaxation and stress reduction, which can help to reduce inflammatory and stress hormone levels. Studies have demonstrated that mindfulness-based therapies can boost general well-being, lower inflammatory markers, and strengthen the immune system.

Yoga and Tai Chi: These practices encourage balance, relaxation, and flexibility by combining physical postures, breathing techniques, and meditation. These methods are useful for controlling inflammation and enhancing general health since they have been demonstrated to lower inflammatory marker levels and boost immune system performance.

Calming Inflammation

Nutrition and Herbal Supplements: Modifying one's diet and taking herbal supplements can help to lower inflammation and maintain immunological balance. When included in a balanced diet or taken as supplements, omega-3 fatty acids, vitamin D, probiotics, and antioxidants like vitamin C and quercetin have all been demonstrated to have anti-inflammatory properties.

Adding Therapies to a Wellness Program

Take into consideration the following actions to successfully integrate holistic therapies into a wellness plan:

Assessment: Consult a medical professional to identify the underlying reasons for your inflammation and your unique demands. Seek advice from a licensed holistic practitioner who can offer customized recommendations based on your unique requirements and preferences, such as an acupuncturist, massage therapist, herbalist, or naturopathic physician.

Customization: Select treatments that suit your needs and way of life. This can entail getting frequent massages, getting acupuncture, or learning stress-reduction techniques. Examine several holistic treatments to see which one is most effective for you. The greatest all-encompassing strategy for reducing inflammation and enhancing well-being can be found in the combination of acupuncture, massage, and mindfulness exercises.

Combine Holistic Therapies with Conventional Treatments: Medication or physical therapy are examples of conventional treatments for inflammation that can be enhanced by holistic therapies. Create a comprehensive wellness plan with your healthcare practitioner that takes into account all facets of your health and combines alternative and traditional therapies. If necessary, combine these therapies with traditional medical care. To effectively manage your treatment, make sure all of your healthcare providers are aware of your holistic approach.

Practice Patience and Consistency: Getting the best outcomes from holistic therapies frequently takes time and dedication. Be kind to yourself and have faith in the process; tiny adjustments done frequently over time can have a big impact on inflammation and general health.

Here are a few success stories and testimonies from people who have benefited from holistic therapy for the control of inflammation to encourage and uplift readers:

"On the advice of a friend, I decided to try **acupuncture** after years of dealing with chronic pain and inflammation. How much relief I felt after only a few sessions astounded me. In addition to relieving my pain, acupuncture made me feel more at ease and in harmony all around."

"**Massage treatment** has significantly improved my ability to manage my arthritic symptoms." My mobility and quality of life have increased, and my joints' inflammation has considerably decreased, thanks to regular massages. I'm

Calming Inflammation

appreciative of my massage therapist's therapeutic touch and the significant positive effects it has had on my health."

"Incorporating mindfulness practices like **yoga and meditation** into my everyday routine has enhanced my mental and physical health." In addition to feeling more collected and at ease, I've also seen a decrease in my inflammatory indicators and an increase in my ability to bounce back from setbacks and stress."

These testimonies are poignant reminders of the deep healing potential of complementary therapies and the significance of managing inflammation holistically. Your body, mind, and spirit may flourish when you embrace holistic ideas and incorporate a range of treatment modalities into your health plan. This will help you live a bright, inflammation-free life.

Calming Inflammation

CONCLUSION

As we draw to a close our exploration of the complexities of inflammation and the range of approaches employed in its management, let's consider the main lessons learned from each chapter:

Understanding Inflammation: An immune reaction that is normal at first but can become harmful when it persists over time is inflammation. The first stage in managing is identifying the symptoms and comprehending the underlying causes.

Immune Balance: Reducing excessive inflammatory reactions requires a healthy immune system. Dietary decisions and lifestyle modifications are important factors in maintaining this equilibrium.

Stomach Wellness: Inflammation is greatly impacted by the state of the stomach. Inflammation can be decreased by maintaining a healthy gut flora with a diet high in fiber and probiotics.

Stress Reduction: Inflammation is exacerbated by prolonged stress. Deep breathing exercises, yoga, and meditation are some techniques that can help control stress and its inflammatory effects.

Anti-Inflammatory Diet: Eating foods high in omega-3 fatty acids and antioxidants can help reduce inflammation. The secret to diet success is moderation and consistency.

Physical Activity: Engaging in regular exercise can help lower inflammation and enhance general health. This includes resistance training, flexibility exercises, and aerobic activities.

Holistic Approaches: A holistic strategy for treating inflammation can be achieved by combining lifestyle changes with integrative therapies like massage and acupuncture.

Although inflammation is a complicated problem, you can manage your health by using a multifaceted strategy that includes holistic therapies, diet, exercise, and stress reduction. Recall that making little, regular changes can result in big gains on the route to well-being.

Use this book as a jumping-off place to explore, try different things, and determine what suits your body the best. Gain knowledge to empower yourself, pay attention to your body, and have patience as you advance. Every move you take to reduce inflammation is a step toward living a better, more energetic life. Your health path is unique to you.

Calming Inflammation

You can control the course of your health. Begin by making one decision at a time starting today, and observe how your body reacts with gratitude and energy.

APPENDIX

Medical and Scientific Terms Glossary

Acute inflammation is the body's temporary immunological reaction to an injury or infection; it manifests as pain, swelling, redness, and heat.

Antioxidants are chemicals that stop other molecules from oxidizing and causing damage to cells.

Chronic inflammation is a long-lasting inflammatory reaction that over time may have a role in the development of many diseases.

Cytokines are tiny proteins that cells release into the environment that specifically affect how cells communicate and interact with one another.

Fish oil contains an omega-3 fatty acid called **eicosapentaenoic acid (EPA)**, which has anti-inflammatory properties.

Unstable atoms known as **"free radicals"** can harm cells, leading to disease and aging.

The complex population of bacteria that reside in the digestive tracts of humans and other animals is known as the **gut microbiome**.

The immune system is the body's line of defense against pathogens and other foreign intruders.

Monounsaturated fats: A kind of fat that is good for you and can be found in avocados and olive oil.

Omega-3 Fatty Acids: Important fats with a host of health advantages, including the ability to reduce inflammation.

Phytonutrients are substances made by plants that offer several health advantages.

Probiotics are live microorganisms that are beneficial to your health, particularly to the health of your digestive system.

One substance found in cruciferous vegetables that has been demonstrated to have anti-inflammatory qualities is **sulforaphane.**

Inflammation that impacts the entire body as opposed to just one area or organ is known as **systemic inflammation.**